From Passion to Purpose: How to Start your own Personal Fitness Training Business

A guide to building a part-time or full-time business as an independent personal fitness trainer and health coach

By

Jack Witt, MS, CPT

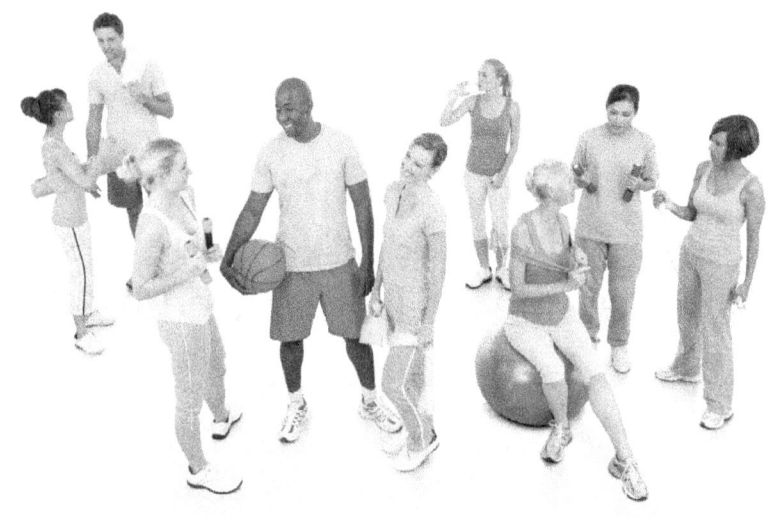

Table of Contents

Part I
Overview of the Fitness Industry- 5

Part II
Personal Fitness Training: Benefits and Rewards 11

Part III
Challenges and Obstacles 15

Part IV
Getting Started 29

Part V
Growing, Learning, and Building your Business..............37

Other
Special Thanks and Dedication 55
About the Author...57
Copyrights 59

1: Overview of the Fitness Industry-Current Trends

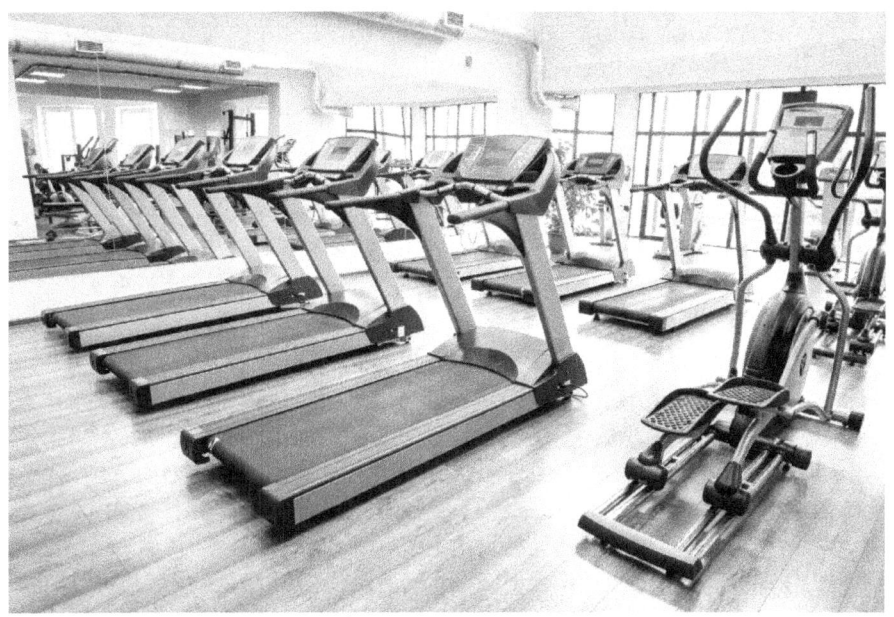

Health Clubs, Personal Fitness Training and Home Exercise

The health and fitness industry is changing and growing at a rapid pace. If you are considering becoming a Personal Fitness Trainer, there is no better time than right now to be a part of this exciting and rewarding career. There were at least 267,000 jobs as certified personal fitness trainers in the U.S. as of 2012, and it's expected to grow at an average pace for all occupations of 13% through 2022 (U.S. Department of Labor). Although the median annual wage for fitness trainers and instructors was $31,720 in May 2012, that takes into account trainers working in clubs like 24 Hour Fitness and Gold's Gym, where the pay is not optimal because the club takes such a large percentage of your hard earned money. But when you start your own business, there's no middle man, and you'll earn much more (although the trade-off is less access to prospects, but we'll cover that in just a while). And, working in large cities as a Personal Trainer, such as Los Angeles (where I live) or New York, where there is greater access to fitness-minded people with higher rates of disposable income, you can easily generate at least double the national average wage and even command upwards of $100 per hour for your private services.

According to the 2014 IHRSA Health Club Consumer Report, health club memberships are near 53 million people, as 18.2% of Americans are Health Club members. The 2013 IHRSA report tells us that 1 out of 5 health club members engage in personal training. The 2012 IHRSA report points out that the total number of health clubs in the USA was almost 30,000, and that a total of 6.4 million Americans used personal trainers in the year 2011. Industry revenues have reached an incredible high of $21 billion and growing.

Age and Exercise

The typical "core" member, who uses their health club an annual minimum of 100 days per year, has the following characteristics (IHRSA 2012):

- Slightly more likely to be male than female

- Average age of 42.9 years
- College graduate or higher
- Average membership tenure of 5.4 years

Most personal training users are between the ages of 25-54 (IHRSA 2012). Although men are more likely to sign up for personal training than women, women are more likely to be frequent users as 43% of female personal training clients engage in at least 11 sessions in comparison with 36% of male clients (IHRSA 2013).

Gender and Exercise

Women are a growing majority of all health club members. The typical private client for wellness coaching is a female over the age of 35 (IHRSA 2007). The rising female membership percentages may be due to the increase in the number of female-only health club facilities, and also the trend towards mind-body-spirit programs and services. Kids are the second fastest growing demographic group in clubs (IHRSA 2007). Youth fitness growth is attributed to the fact that schools are less able to provide physical education programs due to budget cut backs. More children are overweight and have health problems like diabetes, high cholesterol, high blood pressure, low self-esteem, depression and joint/range of motion challenges. The American Heart Association reports that about 1 in 3 children in the United States are overweight or obese.

Income and Exercise

The IHRSA Health Club Consumer Report 2013 shows that more than half of health club members (55%) earn at least

$75,000 in annual household income. Considering that membership is directly correlated to income level, tiered (affordable) membership pricing options may be incredibly valuable to potential members.

Fitness evolving into Wellness

I've noticed the most successful personal fitness trainers go beyond just prescribing exercise and instructions to their clients, they understand how to take it to the next level and act as a life coach and/or wellness coordinator for their clients. The health and fitness industry is growing and evolving and people are searching for deeper meanings and connections, spirituality, mind-body connections, and holistic approaches to their health and living.

It's a very personal relationship that ends up building between you and your clients. Think about it, not too many jobs put you together with your customer or clients 2 to 3 times per week in an intimate setting and space, with personal attention being given each second of the session. The relationship will keep evolving between you and your clients, and it's important to remain professional while also keeping it very personal and connected. Many clients will share their personal lives with you, talk about their past, give their opinions on current events, and want to know more about you personally. It's important for you as the trainer therefore to understand your clients' personality, motivators, stressors, health history, fitness and life goals, and provide them with feedback and support, action plans, steps to success, as well as focus and clarity on reaching their goals. So expanding your continuing education and experience to include life, wellness, and mind-body coaching will certainly be a win-win scenario for you and your clients.

Finally, people all around the world are really starting to "get it" in terms of the importance of wellness and mind-body. But to get in on it and be a wellness coach however requires a deeper understanding of human behavior, motivation, steps to change, as well as the ability to listen, have empathy, and act as a positive and realistic sounding board for your clients.

2: Personal Fitness Training: Benefits and Rewards

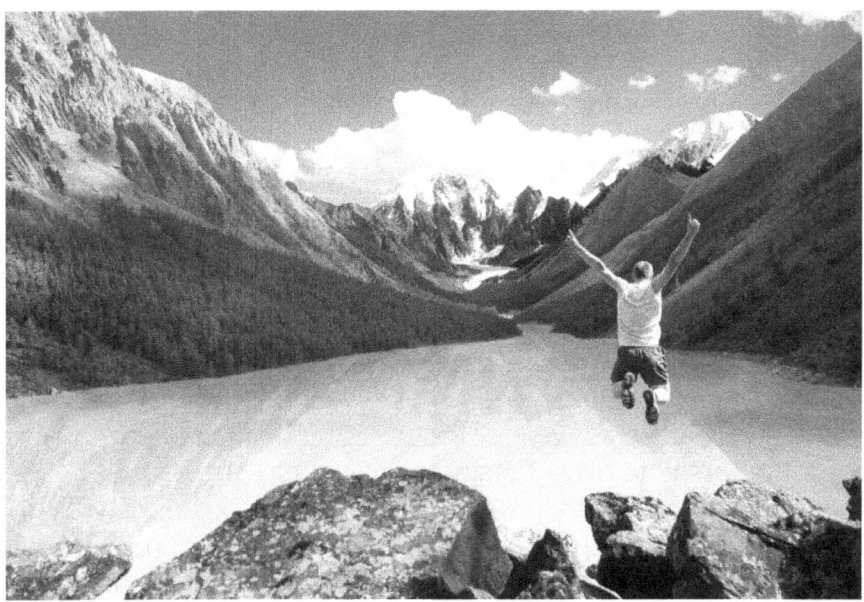

A Passion for what you Do

In my experience in the fitness industry, I've noticed that most personal trainers really enjoy their job. Many come from sports backgrounds and have competed in sports, many come from colleges with physiology degrees, some have worked out on their own body as novices or for contests, and some even come from incredible depths of drug and alcohol addiction and have turned their lives around by concentrating on their health.

11

Some trainers are in their 20's, some are in their 30's, some are in their 40's, 50's etc. Age makes no difference as long as you have a true passion, stay current on your certifications, and believe in your job as a personal trainer. In my case, I didn't become a CPT (Certified Personal Fitness Trainer) until after the events of 9/11 caused me to rethink my corporate sales job that I wasn't feeling totally happy and fulfilled in. No matter where you come from, what your age is, what your past failures or successes are; enjoying what you do to help others achieve wellness, happiness and health is very deeply rewarding.

Control over your Schedule

Don't like working early morning? Can't work evenings due to other obligations? Do you prefer a break in your schedule mid-afternoon to run some errands? As a personal fitness trainer, you have a large degree of autonomy over your schedule. This works well for trainers that work only part-time or for trainers who have outside interests or hobbies that need special attention. However, to build a full time business with optimal revenue, you may need to train on a split schedule, which is what many trainers do. Because many clients like to be trained before they go to work and/or many like to be trained after they get off work in the evenings, a typical split schedule might consist of 6a-10a appointments with an afternoon break and then 5p-9p appointments. In the afternoon you can take a nap, work on expanding and getting more business, or even get caught up on your favorite shows and social media outlets. It's your choice! I do know trainers that simply train from 9a-5p. These trainers decline training early mornings and evenings and find clients that can train only during hours that they are available. Perhaps they have clients who work out on their lunch breaks, or have retired clients that are more flexible to train during afternoons etc. I also know trainers that train all morning, afternoon, and evening. Perhaps they have enormous revenue goals (or enormous mortgage payments). Whatever the case, it's up to you, your budget and lifestyle when you train, and how much you train. Over the years, Sundays became my busiest training day unexpectedly, so I went with it and became known as the "Sunday FundayTrainer".

Helping people live Healthier and Happier

Americans work longer workweeks, eat larger food portions, spend more time in traffic, spend more time in front of computer monitors, eat more fast food and foods with cheap to manufacture high fructose corn syrup, sleep less, and stress more than we did 25 years ago. This has led to an obesity problem. Currently, two thirds of Americans are either overweight or obese. The obesity rate for children has something like doubled in the past 15 years and that's leading to numerous cases of type two diabetes and chronic diseases. As personal fitness trainers and wellness coaches, we have a duty and obligation to bring America back to optimal physical fitness and wellness. Not only can we affect the lives of our clients in this positive way, but also help businesses and organizations reduce costs.

Full Time Pay-Part Time Hours

In a market such as Los Angeles, it is certainly possible and doable to earn "full time pay" working part time hours. At the time of writing this booklet, my current rate is $75 per hour session. I know trainers that charge $100. And, there are some that charge much less. Many "trainers to the stars" charge upwards of $250 per session. An old saying goes, "You're worth as much as somebody will pay you." If you create value, provide great service, motivate, and get results; then that's priceless to people who are improving their wellness and health and living longer and happier lives due to their personal fitness trainer.

Most trainers I know that work part time train about 15-20 sessions per week. Most full time trainers put in as much as 30-50 sessions per week. Some work solely out of one gym or private center, while many "float" around to a variety of private gyms to accommodate their client base. If the latter is the case, commute time is something you should factor in.

3: Challenges and Obstacles

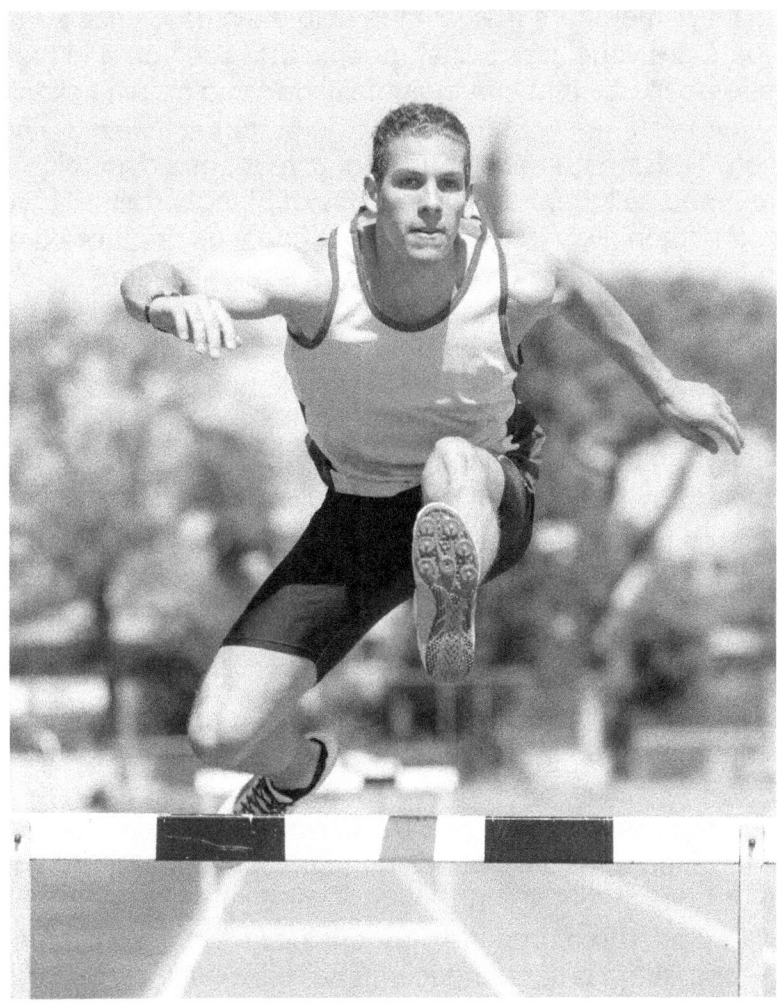

Access to Prospects

I recommend starting off by honing your skills and developing your style working for a fitness center or gym that gets a lot of members that join the club each day. These members are your "prospects", people that see you and that you see each day that can eventually become training clients. Many gyms offer new members a free personal fitness training session. That's a trainer's chance to give them a dynamic workout and sell them on the benefits of hiring a trainer. If you start off immediately in a private gym, chances are there aren't going to be very many prospects to go after since these clubs are mainly just private trainers and their private clients. Most trainers I know start off in a public fitness center like LA Fitness or 24-Hour Fitness, build up a client base, and then at some point make the decision to cut out the middle man and make more money by asking those clients to eventually train at a private gym with them. Most people are loyal to their trainer, not the fitness club. Once that happens, referrals become a major part of your new business. It's important to offer your clients incentives such as free session or two for client referrals. In that meantime, I would recommend joining some organizations to promote your business. Some are strictly for networking, some are designed for leads swapping and some focus on particular industries.

- **Chambers of Commerce**. Chambers of Commerce exist in practically every community in the country. They advocate for local businesses, and can provide you with a platform to promote your business. Check out several chambers before choosing one, they'll usually let you pay a non- member price to attend networking breakfasts, luncheons and mixers. And then if you decide you want to join and maximize your business explore, be sure to attend meetings and events on a regular basis. You won't get immediate clients, it takes a while for people to get to know you and "warm-up". I've had lots of success with the Universal City/North Hollywood Chamber (*www.noho.org*) and the Encino Chamber (*www.encinochamber.org*). I became very active while I was building my business, volunteering on the boards of directors and was even elected President of the Universal City North Hollywood Chamber of Commerce during their Centennial year. It was very rewarding and thrilling, and put my name out there as a professional and credible health and fitness coach.

- **Leads and Networking Groups.** These groups are designed with the idea of providing you with access to other small businesses to which you can promote your business. Some groups only allow one business per category, so you will have no competition for your services within the organization. One of the most popular is LeTip (*www.letip.com*).

- **Service Organizations**. Groups such as the Jaycees, Kiwanis, and Rotary are fun to join to practice volunteerism and get involved in your local community. At the same time, you'll promote your business with people who will become clients, help promote your business, and lead you to other connections in the community that could provide fruitful for your business. Step up and take on a board of directors position and everybody around will eventually know you as the personal fitness trainer. I did this with the Universal City/North Hollywood Jaycees (*www.cajaycees.org*) and it's paid off immensely. The Jaycees are like a

17

worldwide family of young professionals, and even once you "age out" (it's only for 18-40 year olds), you feel like you are still part of the family.

- **Websites & Apps that list and promote you**. There are several companies that have websites and smartphone apps where you can list yourself and your services, either by paying for leads or by paying a commission once somebody books with you. MyTime (*www.mytime.com*) allows you to build a profile for free with pictures and descriptions of your services, and sync your calendar with them so that potential clients can automatically book a time slot and pay up front. You set your own prices and MyTime takes a commission and then pays you via check or direct deposit. Other sites like *www.expect2getfit.com* also don't charge any up- front fees, but will take a commission once you book a client. They simply send you leads in your area, and it's a bit on the trust system, you let them know how much you quoted the client and send them a check for 20% of the first year's revenue with that client. Another site, *www.thumbtack.com* works a little differently. You set up your profile, and you pay for the leads up front, usually in a bundle type package. Like most sites, you set your own prices, and if you get the client, there's no commission that you'll have to pay them since you've already paid for the leads previously. If you do internet/virtual training, *www.wello.com* is a site that connects you with new and existing clients from all over the world where you can conduct sessions and classes with a laptop and web cam from anywhere in the world that you are. They direct deposit payment into your bank account after each session you conduct. I've also known trainers that have had success getting clients on *www.craigslist.com, www.angieslist.com* and *www.meetup.com*. Also, as you get clients from anywhere, have them do a review of you on *www.yelp.com*. Yelp is free to list yourself, but they also do have some upgrade options for a fee that you may want to consider to build up your business.

- **Health Fairs and Run-Walks.** There are a variety of ways to connect with your local community at health-fairs and run-walks. Many schools, colleges, companies, YMCA's and civic groups in your area have annual health fairs that you can be a part of and do fitness assessments, exercise demonstrations, and more. Have a special prize that you are raffling off to create excitement and get people's business cards and contact information for your database. You can even have giveaways at your booth like water, pedometers, tape measures, fit-bands that have your logo and contact information printed on them form product marketing companies such as *http://www.promotionallyminded.com/*. Run-Walks are another terrific place to promote your business and usually have vendor booths. You can even offer to lead a warm up routine for the participants before the race and/or lead stretching for post-race participants. I do this for USC's "Quench the Fire Run", which raises money for chronic pain diseases (www.quenchthefirerun.org/).

- **Your Website and Blog.** For setting up a website, see the section "Sales and Marketing and Social Media" in this book. But a good website that gets traffic driven to it on the web in priceless in terms of access to prospects. I offer a Free Special Report, *"25 Unique*

Ways to make Fitness more Exciting" in exchange for people's contact information, if they sign up for me Free *"Fit Tips Quarterly e-Newsletter"*. That's just one way, so be creative in how you go about it. You might also have a special page on your website that shows all of your social media posts in real time. This helps people connect with you better (literally and emotionally), and keeps them coming back to your website where you sell your products and services.

ACE-certified international fitness professionals (and twins) Alexandra Williams, MA and Kymberly Williams-Evans, MA have been in the fitness industry since the first aerobics studio opened--with them--in Europe, before leg warmers and thong leotards were the rage. Kymberly is former faculty for the Department of Exercise and Sports Studies at University of California Santa Barbara: Alexandra now teaches in that department at UCSB, plus is a freelance editor and writer for IDEA: The Association for Health and Fitness Professionals. Together they own *FunAndFit.org*, a site dedicated to active aging for boom-chicka-boomers. **Here they share with us their Top 10 Tips for Fitness Blogging.**

Just like planning for clients, to be a successful fitness blogger, you must pay attention to the details. You might benefit from these 10 tips that focus on small things that have a big impact.

1. Put your credentials into your profile. There are so many enthusiasts who call themselves experts or gurus. Leave that out and stick with your credentials.

2. Link to research rather than listing it in the middle of your post. If you want to show your sources, put them as footnotes. In print publications, listing resources is required, but when you're blogging, it's a "speed bump" that causes your readers to stop reading.

3. Promote and link to other fitness pros whom you respect. This helps you build a network, credibility, relationships and a higher ranking on Google. If you link to specific posts, they'll get a ping (notification), which increases your chances of having them share or comment on your post. If you link to their home page, they will not be notified.

4. Use your manners. Thank people when they share your posts and tweets. It's also a good idea to ask them to do so, as long as you say please.

5. It's not about you. It never was. It's about your readers. Just like your in-person clients, they are reading and following you because you are offering something they want. Watch your stats to see what's popular and do more of that. Before you write anything, ask yourself, "Who am I writing this for?" Many bloggers are writing for themselves, but you are online to sell a service, so the diary approach isn't really for you (unless your stats say otherwise, in which case ignore this advice).

6. Stay confident with who you are and your area of expertise even when you see other bloggers get big numbers using sensationalism. It's better to have a dedicated niche following than be known for booty or shirtless selfies (though these have their place). Ten dedicated clients pay more than 1,000 voyeurs.

7. If social media truly isn't your thing, outsource it. Hoping it will go away or sort itself out isn't working out too well for the fitness industry. Fitness enthusiasts are all over social media, sharing their personal journeys and advice, while there's a dearth of expert knowledge. Those enthusiasts really do want your information and help.

8. When you're just getting started, pick just one platform so you don't get overwhelmed. Where are your potential clients? Start there.

9. Learn to use hashtags. Just a few go a long way. Except for Instagram. For that, a lot go a long way.

10. Before you pay for expensive programs and services (web, social media, graphics), do a Google or Bing search. Chances are a video already exists with step-by-step instructions.

Getting your Certification

The fitness industry has what seem like a gazillion certifications to choose from. As of the time of the writing of this booklet, there is no governing body that overseas certifications, such as the BAR with the legal profession. Take the time to research your options for which certifications you would like to obtain. Some things Brian Justin from ICTraining points out nicely that you you may want to consider are:

- Reputation in the field of the certifying body and certification.
- The cost of the certification (don't forget to include study materials).
- Exam Locations: Is it feasible for you to get any of the exam session?
- Continued help and support once you have finished becoming certified.
- Renewal Process.

Research the certifications as you would colleges and universities. It is important to be informed so you can make your decision and feel good about it. You may decide to obtain more than one certification so you can gain a different perspective. Since there are many less than credible certifications available, here is a list of the most accepted and reputable ones that are recognized by most major fitness companies that hire trainers such as 24-Hour Fitness, Bally's, and LA Fitness.

- **ACE**-*American Council on Exercise* (www.acefitness.org)
- **ACSM**-*American College of Sports Medicine* (www.acsm.org)
- **AFAA**-*Aerobics and Fitness Association of America* (www.afaa.com)
- **IFPA**-*International Fitness Professionals Association* (www.ifpa-fitness.com)
- **ISSA**-*International Sports Science Association* (www.issaonline.com)

- **NASM**-*National Academy of Sports Medicine* (www.nasm.org)
- **NESTA**-*National Exercise and Sports Trainers Association* (www.nestacertified.com)
- **NSCA**-*National Strength and Conditioning Association* (www.nsca-cc.org)

I would not recommend taking an online certification as your first one. There is no comparison between having an in person teacher demonstrating exercises with correct form and technique in an interactive class, and being able to ask questions and engage your teacher to clearly understand the topic being presented. Places like *www.sochi.edu* (Southern California Health Institute) offer personal trainer courses and classes featuring hands on experience training people. It's a 67.9 quarter credit hours module, but once you graduate, they've teamed up with NASM and you'll receive 6 certifications to start out with. Once you have your certification and have some hands on experience training, online courses can be ideal for continuing education credits which I'll detail later.

After being certified and training in my business for several years, I decided to go back to finish my bachelor's degree and went on to complete my master's degree in Exercise Science. I found the California University of Pennsylvania's (*www.calu.edu*) Global Online program, which was perfect for me, since it was at your own pace, and I could do assignments, cohort online chats, take quizzes and write research papers without it affecting my client base schedule. And living in Los Angeles, I didn't have to spend a minute in traffic, which is the worst in the country. They also teamed up with NASM for the curriculum and I'm happy to say I did it! But again, I would only recommend an online course or degree once you already have hands on experience training people for a good length of time. And also I would recommend a real college (Cal U is a brick and mortar college with 10,000 students that's been around a while and is fully accredited and a non- profit institution).

Motivating and Coaching a Variety of Behavioral Styles

One of the best ways to retain your clients is by adapting your communication approach according to your client's behavioral style. When you tailor your approach and presentation to your client's behavior style you will be able to build rapport and gain acceptance. That's because your behavior style can set up an emotional barrier between you and other people or it can open the door to better communication with them. I suggest learning the 4 core behavior styles of people and how each style likes to be communicated to. It's easy using the DISC method, which is one of the many tools used to measure a person's style. The DISC core styles are:

"D" stands for *"Dominance"*. It's how a person responds to problems and challenges.

"I" stands for *"Influence"*. It's how a person influences others to their point of view.

"S" stands for *"Steadiness"*. It's how a person handles a steady pace.

"C" stands for *"Compliance"*. It's how a person responds to procedures and rules set by others.

First, observe a person's actual behavior (how they act, what they say, and how they say it). Each of these provides a clue that conveys intent.

Now, choose whether a person is "DIRECT and OUTGOING" or "INDIRECT and RESERVED". This will separate the "D"s & "I"s from the "S"s and "C"s in that order.

Then, if you perceived the person as "DIRECT and OUTGOING", you must now decide if they are "MORE COMPETETIVE and DIRECTING", or "MORE TALKATIVE and INTERACTIVE". This separates the "D"s from the "I"s in that order.

Or, if you perceived the person as "INDIRECT and RESERVED", now decide if they are "MORE ACCEPTING and DOING", or "MORE ASSESSING and THINKING". This separates the "S"s from the "C"s in that order.

COMMUNICATION TIPS for each style are:

"D"-Keep your distance, start with business, get to the point quickly, give direct answers, ask for their opinion, strong hand shake.

"I"-Be enthusiastic, allow time for socializing, have fun, use humor, don't be too businesslike or abrupt, don't talk down to them, get close, use gestures.

"C"-Be well prepared, prepare your case in advance, use a straightforward approach, have data to backup your points, don't be disorganized or messy, don't appeal to emotions, don't use gestures.

"S"-Start with personal comments, let them take their time, present your case logically and softly, speak slowly, don't push for quick decisions.

To be more exact and detail oriented, you can have your clients take an Assessment to discover their behavior style. I sell *Lifestyle Insights Reports* to my clients and prospects. They go online and take a quick ten-minute assessment. It produces an 18-page DISC computer generated report of their behavior style and tips and plans for motivating and coaching, ideal environments, communication skills, personal strengths and weaknesses, and more. You can view a sample report on my *Lifestyle Insights* page at *www.getfitwithwitt.com*. There are also paper "scratch off" assessments you can get that will give you and your clients general behavior results. I also encourage you to take your own Behavioral Style Assessment/Profile and discover your strengths and how others perceive you. Contact me and mention you saw this in my book for a 25% discount.

4: Getting Started

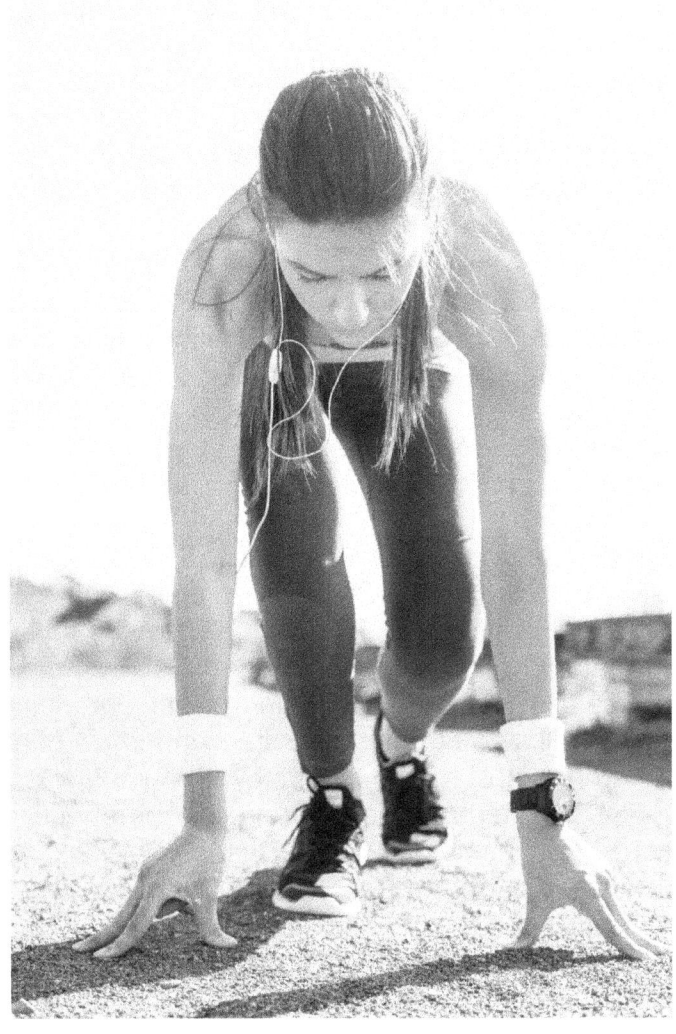

Developing your Business Plan

Personal trainers get so much satisfaction out of their job and have such a passion for helping people achieve health and fitness that they sometimes forget they are running a business. Like any business; bottom line, expenses, taxes, goals, forecasts, and sales and marketing are crucial. Without these practices in place you risk loosing what you have, or not growing beyond what you've got. And, a successful fitness business can reach out to hundreds, thousands, even millions of people to promote health and fitness.

It's important to initially establish and hone your business Vision, Mission, and Core values. This will help you make decisions during tough times and propel you further during prosperous times. A good website to check out for a free simple business plan template is *www.onepagebusinessplan.com*.

I highly recommend a book called "The E-Myth Revisited: Why most Small Businesses Don't Work, and What to do About It." by Michael Gerber. The book dispels the myths surrounding starting your own business and shows how commonplace assumptions can get in the way of running a business. He walks you through the steps in the life of a business -- from entrepreneurial infancy, through adolescent growing pains, to the mature entrepreneurial perspective, the guiding light of all businesses that succeed -- and shows how to apply the lessons of franchising to any business, whether or not it is a franchise. "Small Business for Dummies" -co-authored by Jim Schell and Eric Tyson provides a wealth of strategies for building a winning business. If you've never done sales of any kind, or to just brush up; some good books are "The New Conceptual Selling" and "The New Strategic Selling" by Stephen E. Heiman, Diane Sanchez, and Ted Tuleja.

Insurance

Don't even think about not doing this in today's sue-happy, overly sensitive society. Get proper insurance for your fitness business before training your first client! When fitness professionals think about getting liability insurance, it's usually propelled by the idea of a client suffering an injury and blaming the trainer. But even the safest trainer in the world could eventually end up being sued for more ridiculous reasons, such as not losing weight or achieving the body of their dreams. Or, the lawsuit could be based on perceived sexual harassment; an individual needn't be mentally stable to hire a personal trainer.

When a trainer works for a gym or health club as an employee, the facility itself is covered (or should be covered) with professional liability insurance. But when the trainer is an independent contractor, using the facility's equipment, or training clients in their homes or outdoors, then professional liability insurance will not only cover unexpected legal twists, but will also provide the trainer with peace of mind.

What does professional liability insurance protect you against?

- Claims of injury resulting from inadequate supervision or exercise routines.
- Claims of failing to properly instruct the trainee.

- Claims of improper use or recommendation of equipment.
- Claims of injury resulting from use of substandard equipment.
- Claims that the trainer didn't do something, such as spot the trainee or advise on proper eating.
- Groundless claims, such as accusing the trainer of not being motivating enough.

Most policies limits of liability are in the range of $250,000-$500,000. Annual premiums will cost you in the range of $200-$500.

Source: Publisher Consultant, Inc. (OnFitness Magazine) 2006

Trainer-Client Agreement Forms

Your certification company will most likely have some downloadable forms you can print out to use. The forms will consist mainly of

- Contact Information.
- Terms and Payment.
- Rescheduling, Interruption of Service, and Cancellation.
- Emergency Contacts.
- Informed Consent for Physical Fitness Program and Fitness Testing.
- Liability Waiver.
- Physician Contact Information.
- Health History Questionnaire and Personal Wellness Goals.

You'll want to have each client fill them out completely and sign them and turn them back in to you to keep on file.

CPR

Most gyms and fitness centers will require you to get certified in Cardio Pulmonary Resuscitation. Don't take an online course for this very important knowledge; participate in an interactive class where you get to practice on the training mannequin. The American Red Cross offers local classes that you can take as well as Community Education and Extension Programs at your local community colleges.

Business Entities

Choosing your business structure is just as important - if not more important - than marketing. You should consult with your accountant or your attorney in forming your business. The process in setting up your company is as follows; these are just the key points that need to be done, but not necessarily in the exact order listed.

First, you need to come up with a company name and ascertain if the URL is available for that website. If the URL is available for that name, the next step is to register that name with the Secretary of State in the state that you reside in. At this point, there are two options: One is to consult with your accountant or CPA to decide if you should be a sole proprietor, partnership, limited liability Corporation or a Corporation. At the very least, reserve the name with your Secretary of State for a minimal fee while you decide what business entity you should be.

Here are the four types of business structures and a brief explanation of each:

1. ***Sole Proprietor*** - A Sole Proprietorship is one individual or married couple in business alone. Sole proprietorships are the most common form of business structure. This type of business is simple to form and operate, and may enjoy greater flexibility of management, less legal regulation, and fewer taxes. However, the business owner is personally liable for all debts incurred by the business.

2. ***Partnership*** - A General Partnership is composed of two or more persons (usually not a married couple) who agree to contribute money, labor, and/or skills to a business. Each partner shares the profits, losses and management of the business, and each partner is personally and equally liable for debts of the partnership. Formal terms of the partnership are usually contained in a written partnership agreement.

3. ***Limited Liability Corporation*** - A Limited Liability Company (LLC) is composed of one or more individuals or entities through a special written agreement. The agreement includes: provisions for management, ability to assign interests and distribution of profits and losses. Limited liability companies are permitted to engage in any lawful, for-profit business or activity other than banking or insurance. LLC's cannot have more than 35 shareholders.

4. ***Corporation*** - A Corporation is a more complex business structure. As a chartered legal entity, a corporation has certain rights, privileges and liabilities beyond those of an individual. Doing business as a

corporation may yield tax or financial benefits, but these can be offset by other considerations, such as increased licensing fees or decreased personal control. Corporations may be formed for profit or nonprofit purposes.

Source: American Fitness Professionals and Associates, Inc.

You can get more detailed information on California Business Entities at *www.ss.ca.gov/business*.

5: Growing, Learning, and Building your Business

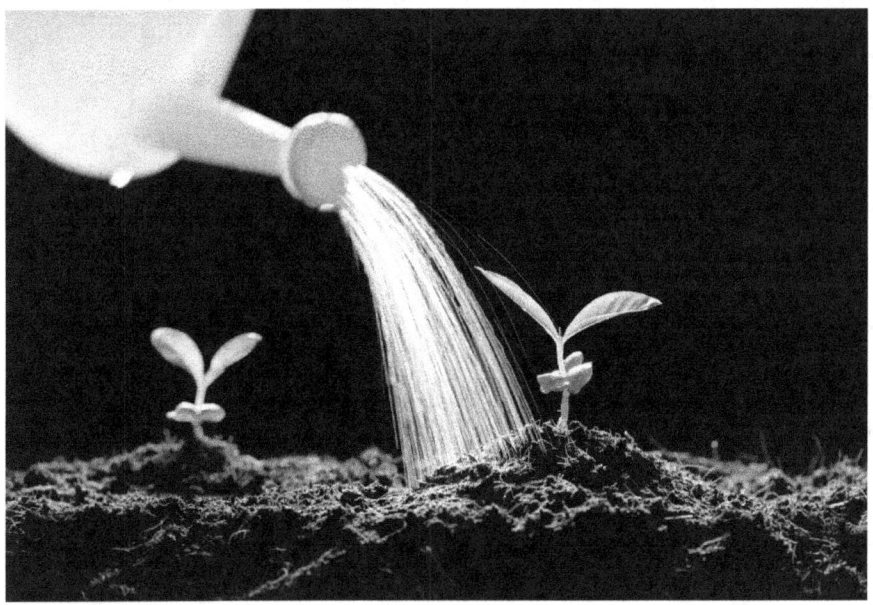

Specialty Training and Continuing Education

Most companies that you will certify with require re-certification each year or every two years. That consists of CEC's (Continuing Education Credits) or also known as CEU's (Continuing Education Units). Typically, these are online or in person classes/workshops you take through your certification company that often consist of specialty areas such as kids or seniors fitness, rehabilitation training, group class instructor, life coaching, plyometrics, sports medicine etc.

Most certification companies will allow you take a certain number of required CEC's outside of their company. For instance, IDEA Health and Fitness Association (*www.ideafit.com*) hosts fitness conferences throughout the United States that offer classes that you can take to gain CEC's to re certify with your certification company. Most certification companies recognize IDEA as a reputable resource for continuing education in the fitness industry. Membership in this organization is about $100 a year and includes monthly fitness journal magazines, access to articles, research and information on their website and more. Other fitness associations include International Health, Racquet, and Sports Club Association (*www.cms.ihrsa.org*).

Setting up a Variety of Revenue Streams (Skype Training, Phone Coaching, Podcasts, Wellness Travel, Books etc.)

Many fitness trainers offer phone coaching and Skype training. Sometimes it's to augment their one-on-one sessions with a client, or it can be ideal for training people who live outside of the area in which you live in who still want your expertise, passion and training style. Selling supplements is also a great way to earn extra income as a personal fitness trainer. However, since there are only so many hours in a day, and you have only so much energy to expend on training clients, it's advantageous to set up passive income: income that you have coming in when you are not physically doing the work. Some prime examples of this are internet-online training, books, DVD's and YouTube channels.

I recently self-published a couple fitness books on Amazon.com (*www.amazon.com/author/jackwitt*). It was free to do and Amazon takes a percentage of the sales. They team up with KDP for e-books (*https://kdp.amazon.com/select*) and CreateSpace (*www.createspace.com*) for paperback books. If you'd like more information on how to do this and some pointers, my personal book coach, Leslie Le Mon has great rates to help first time book authors get through the process of working with Amazon to self-publish. Her email is *les.lemon.author@gmail.com*. And if you need a good proof reader, I recommend mine, Cherrie Higgins at *emailcher@gmail.com*.

An easy way to provide online training sessions for your clients is to buy an inexpensive monthly subscription to sites such as *www.fitnessgenerator.com*. For a small monthly fee you can gain access to thousands of animated in motion exercises with step-by-step instructions to email to clients. Having just one client would pay for itself. I know of trainers who have upwards of 25 online training clients, many who live in other states and possibly other countries.

If clients have a laptop, a desktop with a camera, IPad or just about any device with a camera, they can "Skypercise" with you via *www.skype.com*. I charge $50 per hour to do this and I never leave my home. I instruct them from my desktop or laptop. They don't even need to have a full gym in their home. I encourage them to just purchasing a fit band, some hand-weights, and a Swiss-ball.

As a Personal Fitness Trainer you're the expert, so flaunt it. You can create instructional DVD's and videos. Pod-casts of your workouts or nutritional advise can also be something you can charge a fee for, downloadable from your website. And setting up a free YouTube Channel for your business with a lot of interesting and informative video content can generate lots of views and subscribers and ultimately can earn you money through their "Partner Program".

Do you like to travel and want to earn money in a fitness and wellness environment? SRI International, in partnership with the Global Spa & Wellness Summit, has been measuring the industry annually for the last six years. They report wellness tourism grew to $494 billion in revenues in 2013, a 12.5% increase that's above SRI's original growth forecast of 9%. The report also shows the spa industry grew 58% from 2007 to 2013; in other words, from $60 billion to $94 billion. The number of spas around the globe increased 47%, to 105,591. SRI's report says wellness travel is growing nearly 50% faster than the global tourism overall and represents more than one in seven travel dollars spent worldwide.

I personally love travelling, and have in recent years blended together my love of travel and fitness into a revenue generator: Adventure, Fitness and Wellness Trips. What I do is pick an area in the world where I think people will want to visit, contact local tour operators and work out an agreement where if I bring x number of people I get a free trip, and then earn a commission on the people I bring above the agreed upon amount for the free trip. Most tour operators are more than accommodating. They take the payments directly (that way you don't have to worry about getting a travel agent license, liability insurance and all the costs and overhead of owning a travel agency) and you become sort of their sales person and the group leader/organizer. I've led several successful fitness and adventure domestic trips to various state and national parks, and internationally to places like Costa Rica (through *www.costaricantrails.com*) and Peru/Machu Picchu (through *www.ZephyrAdventures.com*), and Jordan and Israel and Palestine soon (through *www.otbtravel.com/).* If you think this is something you'd like to try as an additional revenue stream, my *"Fit Travel Partners"* group is always looking for amiable and people friendly trainers that like to travel and are good with diverse groups of people. Contact me today to learn more about up-coming trips that you can be a group leader on.

Entrepreneur Basics

Having your own small business obviously takes hard work and dedication. Don't be surprised if you feel like it's a 24/7 commitment, because a lot of time it takes that kind of focus and determination to succeed and beat the competition. Kinesiology and exercise science are one of the fastest growing majors in colleges today, so you're going to have a lot of competition. Working smarter will give you the edge to succeed. **I've asked Susan Baker, Owner of Escape Hatcher (*www.escapehatcher.com*) , a company that helps people just like you create, plan and enjoy their dream "solopreneur" jobs, to give 5 tips from her 5 M's (Mindset, Mission, Monetization, Marketing & Mechanix). Here's her advice for you:**

My "escape plan" hatching program takes my clients through the 5 "M" modules which I've found are essential for solopreneurial success: Mindset, Mission, Monetization, Marketing & Mechanix, for budding fitness gurus, I think incorporating some sound practices from all areas is sure to help you succeed.

#1 Mindset - Nothing happens without a strong mindset foundation. One of the areas that will definitely yield results is to continually inf"YOU"se your business with you...spend time really deciphering what you excel at and what will make your ideal client want to work with you. A consistent practice of checking in, extracting your awesomeness and defining what makes you YOUnique is essential for any solopreneur who wants to set themselves apart. You'll make it easier for your target market (aka your peeps) to find you and that is ALWAYS a good thing. This also builds confidence (which you will need oodles of along the way). If you can't see this clearly, get outside of yourself and attempt to see yourself through the eyes of people who see it all the time ... i.e. family members, friends, colleagues, networking buddies, etc.

#2 Mission - As a solopreneur it's not enough to be pursuing $$$ only, it's my firm belief that you need to be on a mission to truly succeed. It' what will get you up in the morning, from point A to point B and keep you going during the challenging early stages. Sure, every business wants/needs to make money, but it's the mission that will propel you the furthest the fastest. Find yours. What do you want to achieve? Who do you want to help? Why does this matter to you? What is your story and how does it inform the formation of your business? Figure this out because you will need to know this to market yourself, to communicate with your potential clients and to build your brand.

#3 Monetization - Come up with a monetization strategy that expands beyond your core product/service. You don't want to be in a position of relying on ALL of your income from one source. Spread the love. You also don't want to bite off more than you can chew, so start with 2-3 in the 5 most commonly utilized monetization arenas: minutes for money (coaching, training, projects hired by time, etc.), leveraged (workshops, classes, webinars, etc.), passive (e-books, on line courses, kits, DIY programs, etc.), continuity (member sites, subscriptions, etc.), products (existing products you can brand).

#4 Marketing - Get used to the idea that in the beginning you should expect to spend about 85% of your time marketing and embrace Pareto's Principle early on. (20% of your efforts will yield 80% of your results)...so analyze often to see what is working, expand on what works, and ditch what doesn't after a fair amount of time. My recommendation is to pick 2-3 marketing vehicles that appeal to you that you think you will be good at and go really deep with those, instead of trying to spread yourself too thin and try every new hot on line marketing method.

#5 Mechanix - Don't allow yourself to fall into the trap of getting bogged down with things like building your websites, or filing for your biz license and things like this - these things are usually VERY easy and just require some focused work. There are SO MANY bootstrappy resources for solopreneurs these days...even something like getting a simple website up with just a few pages is incredibly easy with a tool like Weebly with their drag/drop functionality. There are other options as well, but you can literally build a nice looking website in about 10 minutes there, publish it and be live. Over the years that I've been working with clients, this area is hands down the place where people get tripped up the most...if you find that no matter how hard you try this is happening to you, it's often well worth the $$$ to outsource these things with a business savvy VA or a trusted friend who thrives in this arena...

I hope some of this is helpful! I'm looking forward to hearing more about your journey.

Sales and Marketing and Social Media.

If you're not proactive in obtaining new clients by constantly seeking new clients through sales and marketing efforts...well I don't have to tell you what is going to happen. You'll have a small group of clients you'll train, some will not continue, some may get sick, some may reach their goals and stop, and some may take long breaks or vacations that'll make paying your bills tough. I've found that being an independent trainer, there's always going to be at least a 20% turnover ratio, so you've always got to be pro-active for new clients. I talked a little about the importance of joining networking organizations. But let's take it a few steps further.

The first thing I would recommend is establishing a website. It makes you more credible, and it provides a place for you to sell your training products and services, and collect contact information from viewers. For beginners, I would recommend a "build it yourself" templated site that will allow you to customize templates that are already set up with your own logos, pictures, and text. The "Website Builder" option through *www.sadaweb.com* runs as low as $10 per month. It's a great value and easy to understand and use. There are plenty of free one page website builders out there like Wordpress (great for blogs, small to medium-sized websites of all kinds), Drupal (great for medium to large-sized websites),

Webs, Angelfire, Google Sites, Webnode, Wikia (great for wikis) where you can get started without breaking the bank. Decide what the name of your site is going to be and reserve that name at *www.sadaweb.com*. It shouldn't cost you more than $15 per year. They also do web hosting.

As you grow your business and your website needs to become more visible and accessible, you'll want more pages and functionality; therefore, you'll want to find a good, creative, reliable Webmaster to design and build a quality site for you and make updates to it. I recommend Carol Manooglan. She's based out of the UK, but wherever you are in the world, she can take your ideas and goals and build a super great looking website that functions optimally and easily for your business needs. She can be reached at *carolmanooglan@msn.com*.

Writing and sending out a Fitness Tips Newsletter (I use *www.icontact.com*) is a great way to get new clients and help retain existing customers. Keep a good database of contacts and send out a newsletter monthly, or even every two weeks. It'll give you top of mind awareness and position you as the expert in your field. They say it takes people up to 7 times of seeing your company's name in either an ad, email, postcard, book, TV to buy your product or service. Another way to get new clients is to write articles pro bono for local papers or websites. I've been writing fitness and health tips for a local website in my area called *www.nohoartsdistrict.com* and get almost 1,000 reads per month now. You can post your articles on Yahoo Voices, submit a couple sample articles to *www.examiner.com* and they may hire you to write fitness, health and wellness articles for your local area. The possibilities are limitless really, just do your research and determine if you need to be "exclusive" with whatever site or blog you are writing articles for. It's best not to be at first, so you can re-post your articles to several different sites for maximum efficiency.

Check out *www.30minutearticles.com* for help and guidance on writing articles. Call up the person in charge of the health or fitness section of a paper, magazine or website and ask them if they are looking for articles that might be of interest to their readers. Tell them you'll write articles for free for posting your contact information. Some websites will also let you do this, try contacting *www.bodybuilding.com* or *www.ezinearticles.com*. There are services like *www.submityourarticles.com* that will submit to numerous websites for a small monthly fee to save you time. Blogs are a great way to generate interest in your products and services and engage people in general on the internet. You can set up a free blog at *www.blogger.com*, which is owned by Google.

And now I'm going to try to give you and overview of social media and how to use it for your fitness and health business, knowing full well I'm not by any means close to being any kind of expert and knowing that by the time I publish this book, things will have evolved anyway. But yes you can certainly utilize social media to build your business and retain existing clients: YouTube Channel, Twitter, Facebook, LinkedIn, Tumblr, Instagram, Pinterest, Google +, Vine, etc. are the main ones. I recently attended the Fit Social Conference (*www.fitsocialconference.org*) in Colorado and it brought together hundreds of bloggers and social media enthusiasts for the fitness and health industries. One of the workshops/classes was "Overview of Social Media" by *www.room214.com*. **Stacey and Maya were the dynamic presenters of this workshop, and I've asked them to**

provide a basic overview of Social Media tips and strategies for the fitness industry. Here it is:

Social media can present a huge opportunity for any start-up company, especially in the fitness industry. Social offers the perfect opportunity to establish a unique brand presence that differentiates you from the competition. Creating buzz around your brand with social requires little to no cost to implement up front, but can have great financial returns. Social media is the perfect place to connect with current customers, find new ones, and turn people into brand advocates.

In order to have the most successful presence on social, it is essential to know your audience. Look at which networks your target audience uses on a daily basis. Do some investigating and ask your current customers where they are spending the most time online. Once you determine what networks are the best, only join one or two to begin with so you can concentrate on making these networks the best and most engaging. Establish a strong fan base before adding a new network to your roster.

Help your content be and stay relevant by thinking about who you're speaking to. What do they want to know and why should they read your content? Mix it up and don't be afraid to post off-topic every so often as long as it is fresh and relevant. Posts around new music, shows or awards, for example, draws in your audience and makes your brand human and relatable. Develop a brand voice or persona that all of your posts embody. Is it funny, straight-talking, or sarcastic? All posts should help build the tone of your company and let your audience know what your business personality is like. Keep an eye on the posts that have the highest engagement (likes, comments, shares) and tailor your content based on this insight.

It takes commitment to grow your social networks and drive engagement. Links are key: always include links back to your blog or website, and track referrals and conversions with a tool like Google Analytics. Try to have a real conversation with your customers. The brands that are doing social media best are the ones interacting and answering questions in real time. This lets the brand appear genuine and engaged.

Determine your own definition of success and set goals accordingly. Analytics are useful to measure traffic and website views. Keep track of conversions such as sales or newsletter sign ups and attendance at events. As your business grows it might be time to invest in professional strategy, management or reporting. Consider Room 214 for any of these social or digital needs and in the meantime, check out Room 214's top three tips for each of these social networks:

Facebook
1. Post 3-4 times per week with pictures
2. Use Facebook insights to determine which content your fans consume most
3. Use visuals as much as possible and keep the copy short and sweet

Instagram
1. Post 2-3 times per week
2. Make photos colorful and engaging with short text
3. Use videos to show parts of workouts

Twitter
1. Post 4-5 times per day, including retweets of influencers
2. Create and use hashtags strategically
3. Place links in tweets and/or pair with pictures

Pinterest
1. Curate your own content. Use in-house production to film your own videos or take photos of workout tips or fitness inspiration.

2. Edit all posts to link back to your home page so you're driving traffic in the right direction

3. Certify your site through Pinterest to gain credibility and promote business

Google+
1. Google+ is an important social network to utilize for Search Engine Optimization (SEO) purposes

2. Re-purpose content from other networks on Google+

3. Try a content publisher like Sprout Social or HootSuite to schedule across multiple networks at once.

For more social media tips, visit *www.room214.com.*

If you're comfortable public speaking, then a great way to promote yourself and your business is to speak at schools, churches, community groups, etc. on fitness and health. People are always really interested in learning about the latest diet tips and training techniques. Be sure to get everybody's contact information for your database that you're building for marketing purposes. If you're not comfortable speaking in front of groups contact your local toastmasters at *www.toastmasters.org*.

Another great way to get new clients is to establish rapport and relationships with local chiropractors, doctors, dentists, and health professionals. Give them a free session or two so that they can recommend you to their clients. Ask them if you can put your brochures and/or business cards in their offices. Don't forget to be creative! Contact spas and massage professionals to work out a referral program, post on *www.craigslit.org*, and send Press Releases when you get a speaking engagement or have a unique success story with a client. A very good website that gives in depth tips and examples on many of the sales and marketing ideas I've been talking about is *www.publicityhound.com*. Register for their free weekly e-blast, it is chock-full of ideas that can translate into your fitness business. Also, *www.keuilian.com* has several products and services specific to the fitness industry for promoting your fitness business. (And of course I'm available for one-on-one customized consultation and planning on attracting new clients and setting up a successful long-term fitness and wellness business model.)

Getting through Slow Periods

Celebrity Personal Trainer, Nancy Sexton of *Realife Fitness* shares with us now some good advice and encouragement on how to stay positive and focused during dips in business. Every business experiences good prosperous times and leaner slower times. It's important that you anticipate and handle your slow periods in a well-planned and positive fashion.

Avoiding Slow Times: In the world of Personal Training (PT), there are busy times, and there are slow times, it's just the nature of the beast. That's why it's so important to keep a slow and steady pace with your promotion and advertising. During a spike in business, it's easy to overlook promotion and advertising, because, well, you're booked, but that is the precise time that you should be really beating the drum for business.

Why?

Because potential clients want to work with busy trainers, and you want to create an energy around your business that breeds more business. i.e.: "Nancy is amazing, but call her right away, I know she is really busy." "She is the best, hopefully you can get on her schedule." Versus the slow business energy, i.e.: "Call her, and see if she'll swing you a deal, I know she can use the money." "She's never very busy."

It is far better to have a waiting list of people who want to train. Chances are they won't even think about asking for a deal, they'll just be glad that you got on your schedule.

How To Get Out Of A Slump:

1. First, change your attitude and your verbiage. Don't talk about being slow, talk about how you are going to get new clients. Don't talk to your existing clients about your financial problems, tell them how excited you are for new clients. A good tool to help change how you deal with the lack of clients is called EFT tapping, check it out YouTube. Works for me, every time.

2. Use your slow periods to update your website, Facebook page, Yelp, Twitter, YouTube or Instagram. Work on a blog and link it to your other pages. Pre-load future posts to your social media management with apps like HootSuite, TweetDeck or Seesmic. Pre-loading posts will keep you cool during busy times.

3. Ask your clients to post a review on FB or on Yelp or where ever your business is listed.

4. Do not dwell on being slow. If you stay focused on getting more clients, you won't even have time to think about it.

5. Create a trailer for you and your business that you can use to promotion. Keep it between 20-30 seconds and really grab the viewer's attention within the first 5 seconds. Then utilize it on every site that you can find. Make sure that it also contains your contact info and your website.

6. Use the down time to get yourself into even better shape. Don't be a lazy fat trainer. Be an example not a peer.

7. Be social! You can't expect everyone to find you. Get out into the world looking and feeling fantastic, and always carry business cards.

8. Be active with your community. Volunteer, join the Chamber of Commerce, talk to local Youth Groups, get involved and help others. This helps to keep people talking about you. And it's good energy.

9. Do not be afraid to spend money to make money. And don't be afraid to offer new clients a free consultation session, if they are interested in it. Approach it from this angle. "I give the consultation for free, because you shouldn't have to spend money to see if we are going to be a good fit for each other." Immediately the client knows that you are smart, considerate and that you are concerned for their well being. Consultations can be done over the phone, but I like to do them in person. It's basically my time to shine and it also allows me to up sell my packages.

10. Be prepared. Slow times or lack of money can happen for many reasons, especially if clients purchase large packages. A wind fall of money today can make for penny pinching later. Figure out a good system for managing your money and let it work for you.

Training YOUniquely

Every business needs to find a niche market, and identity, something unique about it that separates it from other businesses with the same product or service. I suggested earlier discovering your behavior style and how others perceive you. Taking that a step further into branding your own unique identity and personality as a trainer can give you an edge. There are all types of trainers: Quiet Trainers, Loud Trainers, Humorous Trainers, Big Trainers, Small Trainers, Slim Trainers, Chubby Trainers. Not one type is better than the other. But, the most successful trainers are the ones that stand out from the others. Therefore, exam who you are at heart and what your strengths are, your core values…and practice being that person as a trainer all the time, in a professional manner. Carve out your own unique identity as a trainer. Is it the type of clothes you wear? Is it the type of questions you ask during a training session? Is it your session lengths or your pricing options? Next, I suggest keeping a record of your successes with clients and the types of workout programs and exercises that you used to achieve these successes. Was there some type of technique you used that was unique? Was there something that you did that not many other trainers do that makes your training techniques unique and brings results to your clients? If so, document it and now you have your unique training styles and/or techniques.

The most important thing I'd like to close with is to make sure to have fun being a personal fitness trainer. If, after a while of working as a personal fitness trainer, you are still not sure it's a perfect match for you, or you're not getting immense satisfaction and fulfillment out of your job....change direction and do something else. Your life is too important not to be earning a living doing what you really enjoy, what really motivates you and inspires you. Find your inner voice, your calling, and your greatness. Shine your light! Engage in work that taps your talent and your passion, and you can live a very meaningful, successful, and happy life.

From all of us here that have written and contributed to this book, we wish you a very successful and abundant career as a Personal Fitness Trainer and Wellness Coach.

And as I like shout out in the gym with my clients; "Wooh Hooh!!!"

Jack Witt, MS, CPT, Lifestyle Fitness Coach
"Get Fit with Witt" | 818-760-3891 | Jack@getfitwithWitt.com

Special Thanks and Dedication

Adisorn "Tan" Toonsap- Book cover design.

Leslie Le Mon - for her continuing coaching, feedback and support on the continuing journey of writing and publishing my book(s). Email her at les.lemon.author@gmail.com as she is always happy to consult with writers, first-time or otherwise.

Cherie Higgins - for proofing the book(s).

Greg Highley - for my personal photographs.

Rony Armas & Agnes Avagyan - for the cartoon Jacks.

International Health, Racquet & SportsClub Association (IHRSA).

Carrie Spencer - for Webmastering www.GetfitwithWitt.com.

The personal fitness training gyms that I've worked with over the years, including *BodyImage, AtOne Fitness, BodyUSA, Shape It,* and *Knuckles.*

Some of the other super great fitness trainers I've had the opportunity to work on community and charity projects with over the years - *Nancy Sexton, Steven Greene, Lisa Smith* and *Wendie Wilson.*

All of my personal fitness training clients throughout the years who have been so supportive of me and with whom many I've become good friends with: *Stefanie, Lisa, Ilene & Jim & Sylvia, Alda, Kara & both Davids, Eric, Cookie, Erwin, Mark, Youchanan, Jim, Betsy, Anna, Tanya, Paulina, Selenne, Sonia, Annie!, Kirk, Aliki, Leanne, Jeanne, Jane & Keith, Tony & Lana, Sheila, Gloria, Elizabeth, Lisa, Ellen* and *Elaine, Lisa* and *Nancy* and *Jessica, Jane & Dorain, Susan, Emily, Thang & Nancy, Paul, Lou, David, Sean, Kimberly, Annie, Kevin, Scott, Stacy* and *Matt, Phil, Elaine (Ink), Stephanie, King, Donna, Michael, Jaime* and *Jackie, Chris, CherylAnn, Stuart &Robin, Jane & Dorain, MaryLu, Karen & Karen & Andreas, Roz, Ricky, Beneranda, Mayra, Breanna, Sylvia, Mojgan, Patricia, Gina & Dezi & Anna, Bill, Marlene & Chris, Roni* and *Tess, Stuart & Robyn, Zaven, Justin, Kristie, LuLu, Trudy, Howard, & Jenny.*

Expert contributors to this book: Alexandra Williams & Kymberly Williams-Evans of FunandFit.org, Susan Baker of EscapeHatcher.com, Stacey Kawakami and Maya Shaff from Room214.com, and Nancy Sexton of RealifeFitness.com .

About the Author

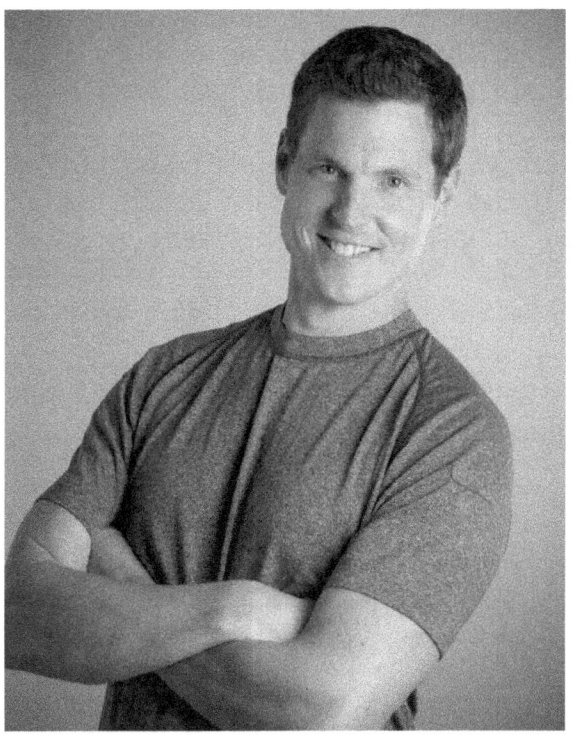

Jack Witt is a Health & Fitness Coach and Active Travel Guide, based out of Los Angeles since 2003. He holds a Master's Degree in Exercise Science, and is a healthy community organizer, serving as past President of the Universal City North Hollywood Jaycees (Junior Chamber) and Chamber of Commerce. His awards include "Outstanding Young Californian", "Angel" and "Small Business of the Year."

57

He is an NASM Certified Personal Fitness Trainer and TTI Certified Behavioral Analyst. His public speaking and workshop engagements include Los Angeles Unified School District, Social Security Administration, Volunteer League of the San Fernando Valley, and Los Angeles Valley College. Jack has worked with kids, adults and seniors, helping all of them take charge of their health and wellness.

Jack enjoys organizing domestic and international *Active Travel Trips* for groups, which include nature walks and day hikes to spiritual and sacred places.

Visit Jack's website at: www.GetfitwithWitt.com

Friend Jack on Facebook at https://www.facebook.com/jack.witt.186

Follow Jack on Twitter / Instragram @GetfitwithWitt

Watch Jack's YouTube Channel www.youtube.com/user/getfitwithWitt

Check out Jack's other books at www.amazon.com/author/jackwitt

Copyrights

All content, illustrations, images and photos in *From Passion to Purpose: How to Start your own Personal Fitness Training Business,* including the cover design; are created by, property of, and copyrighted by Jack Witt © 2015. Some photos and images licensed through Fotolia.